Overcoming Depression: *Finding Hope In The Face of Depression*

I have seen friends sink deeper into depression and fail to make it through. As painful as it was that despite all the help we gave, we were too late! I don't want it to be your story too. Take heed while there is still time and change a life!

--------------Let's make the difference--------------

Dedication

To my FATHER Vitalis and MOTHER Roseline. Thank you for your unwavering support during the worst periods of my life. I sincerely appreciate and will never forget what your comfort meant.

Foreword

Depression, a complex and pervasive mental health condition, affects millions of lives worldwide. At our core, we believe that understanding depression is the key to overcoming it. Depression transcends mere sadness. It engulfs individuals in a relentless cycle of despair, robbing them of motivation and joy.

Depression wears many masks, making it essential to recognize its varied symptoms. From persistent feelings of hopelessness and fatigue to changes in appetite and sleep patterns, depression manifests both physically and emotionally. Understanding these signs empowers individuals and their support networks to intervene early, fostering a swifter path to recovery.

Dr. Richard Wambua (PhD, Psychology)

Preface

Depression, a silent and often misunderstood battle, affects millions of lives around the world. It creeps into the mind like a shadow, robbing individuals of their joy, motivation, and zest for life. But here's the undeniable truth: Depression does not define you, and you can overcome it.

In the pages of this book, "Overcoming Depression: You Can Get Whole Again," we embark on a journey of healing and transformation. Depression, with its suffocating grip, may have brought you to your knees, but it doesn't have to keep you there. This book is your guiding light, your lifeline, and your roadmap to rediscovering the joy, purpose, and fulfillment that depression has stolen from you.

Contents

Chapter 1:

Understanding the Depths of Depression

Some physical health conditions can mimic depression symptoms. It's essential to consult a healthcare professional to rule out any underlying medical causes.

D epression often makes you feel like you're navigating uncharted waters with no compass, no map, and no hope. It's crucial to start this journey by understanding what depression truly is and how it affects your life.

Depression is not simply feeling sad or down for a few days. It's an intricate web of emotions, thoughts, and physical sensations that can persist for weeks, months, or even years. It's the weight that drags you down when you try to get out of bed in the morning. It's the voice in your head that tells you you're worthless, that life is meaningless, and that happiness is an unattainable dream.

Let's delves deep into the different facets of depression, from its emotional toll to its physical manifestations

Types of Depression: Understanding the Many Faces of this Silent Struggle

In today's fast-paced world, it's essential to understand that depression is not a one-size-fits-all condition. It manifests in various forms, affecting individuals in unique ways. To navigate this complex topic, we delve into the different types of depression, shedding light on the nuances and challenges that each subtype presents. This chapter provides you with a comprehensive understanding of depression, enabling you to recognize the signs and seek the right support when needed.

Major Depressive Disorder (MDD)

Major Depressive Disorder, commonly known as clinical depression, is perhaps the most well-known type of depression. It is characterized by persistent feelings of sadness, hopelessness, and a loss of interest or pleasure in activities. MDD can significantly impact daily life, making even the simplest tasks seem insurmountable. It often requires a combination of therapy and medication to manage effectively.

Persistent Depressive Disorder (PDD)

Persistent Depressive Disorder, formerly known as dysthymia, is a form of depression that lingers for an extended period, typically lasting for at least two years. People with PDD experience low energy, self-esteem issues, and difficulty concentrating. While the symptoms may not be as intense as MDD, their chronic nature can be equally debilitating.

Bipolar Disorder

Bipolar Disorder is characterized by extreme mood swings, cycling between manic and depressive states. During manic episodes, individuals may feel excessively elated, impulsive, and full of energy. Conversely, depressive episodes bring about the classic symptoms of depression. Effective management often involves mood stabilizers and therapy to balance these extreme shifts.

Seasonal Affective Disorder (SAD)

Seasonal Affective Disorder is a unique type of depression that occurs with the changing seasons, most commonly during the fall and winter months. Reduced exposure to sunlight can disrupt the body's internal clock, leading to symptoms like fatigue, oversleeping, and weight gain. Light therapy and lifestyle adjustments can be effective in treating SAD.

Postpartum Depression

Experienced by some new mothers, Postpartum Depression is triggered by hormonal changes after childbirth. It can manifest as intense sadness, anxiety, and difficulty bonding with the newborn. Seeking prompt treatment and support is crucial for the well-being of both the mother and the child.

Psychotic Depression

Psychotic Depression is a severe form of depression that includes symptoms of psychosis, such as delusions or hallucinations. Individuals with this condition often struggle with distinguishing between reality and their distorted perceptions. Antidepressant medications combined with antipsychotic drugs are typically used in treatment.

Atypical Depression

Atypical Depression is characterized by symptoms that differ from the classic signs of depression. These individuals may experience increased appetite, weight gain, excessive sleep, and extreme sensitivity to rejection. It often responds well to psychotherapy and certain antidepressant medications.

Situational Depression

Also known as adjustment disorder with depressed mood, Situational Depression occurs as a response to a specific life event, such as the loss of a loved one, a divorce, or a job loss. It usually subsides as the individual adapts to the new circumstances, but counseling can be beneficial during this challenging period.

Premenstrual Dysphoric Disorder (PMDD)

PMDD is a severe form of premenstrual syndrome (PMS), characterized by severe mood disturbances, irritability, and physical symptoms in the days leading up to menstruation. Hormonal treatments and lifestyle changes can help manage PMDD.

Substance-Induced Mood Disorder

Substance abuse can lead to depression-like symptoms, which can persist even after the substance is no longer used. Treatment often involves addressing both the substance abuse and the underlying depressive symptoms.

Depression is not a monolithic condition but a multifaceted one with various types, each presenting its unique challenges. Recognizing the type of depression one is facing is the first step toward effective management and healing. If you or someone you know is struggling with depression, seeking professional help is crucial. Understanding these different types of depression helps you offer them the support and resources necessary to overcome this silent struggle. Also, it better equips you to seek help and embark on a path toward recovery.

In the upcoming chapters, we'll explore the transformative power of mindset, the importance of seeking professional help, and the strategies and techniques that can guide you toward a life free from the shackles of depression. Remember, this is your journey, and with the right knowledge and support, you can emerge from the darkness into a life filled with hope, purpose, and happiness.

Chapter 2

How do you know you are depressed? – What are the signs?

Depression can affect people of all ages and genders. It doesn't discriminate.

Depression is like the "invisible enemy," it can sneak into your life without you even realizing it. It's not just about feeling a little down or blue; it's a complex emotional state that can engulf your entire world. But how do you know you are depressed? What are the signs that you should be aware of? The chapter delves deep into the labyrinth of depression, shedding light on its elusive signs and providing you with the tools to recognize them. So, grab a cup of tea, get comfy, and let's embark on this journey to understanding the intricate language of depression!

The Whispering Shadows of Depression

Persistent Sadness or 'The Blues' That Won't Go Away

- You find yourself feeling persistently sad, down, or low for weeks on end.
- Even activities that used to bring you joy no longer do.
- Life seems colorless, and you can't seem to shake off that heavy feeling in your chest.

The Tiresome Tug of Fatigue

- You wake up tired and go to bed tired.
- No amount of sleep or rest seems to rejuvenate you.
- Daily tasks that used to be easy now feel like climbing a mountain.

The Weight of Guilt and Worthlessness

- Guilt and worthlessness haunt your thoughts.
- You feel like a burden to others.
- Your inner critic never takes a break, constantly berating you.

A Foggy Mind and Poor Concentration

- Your mind feels like a foggy day, making it hard to concentrate.
- Simple decisions become monumental tasks.
- Forgetfulness becomes your unwelcome companion.

Changes in Appetite and Weight

- You experience significant changes in appetite—either overeating or losing interest in food.
- Your weight starts fluctuating rapidly without any deliberate changes in diet or exercise.

The Isolation Abyss

The Desire to Withdraw from Social Life

- You start avoiding social gatherings and close friends.
- Even simple conversations become exhausting.
- Isolation feels like a refuge.

Trouble Connecting with Loved Ones

- Your relationships start to strain.
- You can't seem to communicate your feelings to those close to you.
- Loneliness creeps in even when surrounded by people.

Escaping into a Digital World

You find solace in escaping into the digital realm, like social media or video games.

These become coping mechanisms to numb the pain.

Real life starts to feel disconnected and overwhelming.

The Sleepless Nights and Restless Days

Insomnia or Hypersomnia

- You struggle with insomnia, unable to fall asleep or stay asleep.

- Alternatively, you find yourself sleeping excessively, unable to get out of bed.

Early Morning Awakening

- You wake up much earlier than intended, often accompanied by racing thoughts.
- Mornings become a battleground of anxiety and despair.

The Vicious Cycle of Sleep and Depression

- Lack of sleep worsens your depression.
- Depression worsens your sleep problems, creating a never-ending cycle.

The Physical Manifestations of Despair

Aches and Pains with No Apparent Cause

- Unexplained physical aches and pains become frequent.
- Medical tests often yield no clear cause.

Recurring Headaches or Digestive Problems

- Persistent headaches or digestive issues become part of your daily life.
- Stress and depression seem to manifest physically.

The Dark Pull of Self-Harm or Suicidal Thoughts

- You contemplate self-harm or even suicide.
- These thoughts are not fleeting but persistently haunt your mind.
- Seeking help becomes crucial at this stage.

While some individuals may experience temporary relief from depression, it often requires treatment, therapy, or medication to fully recover. Encourage open communication, offer your support, and suggest seeking professional help. Be patient and understanding

Chapter 3

The Power of Mindset: Overcoming the Darkness

A journey of self-discovery and growth

In the realm of battling depression, where the storm clouds of despair seem relentless, one weapon stands out as a beacon of hope: mindset. We, as warriors in this battle against depression, understand that it's not just about the chemical imbalances in our brains or the external challenges we face. It's about the way we perceive, react, and ultimately, conquer the darkness that engulfs us. In this chapter we delve deep into the transformative power of mindset and how it can lead us from the depths of depression into the radiant light of resilience.

Recognizing the Battle Within

Depression is often compared to a relentless storm, clouding our thoughts, sapping our energy, and leaving us feeling helpless. To rise above this tempest, we must first acknowledge that we are in a battle—a battle against our own minds. We must understand that it's not a sign of weakness to seek help or to admit that we are struggling. It's a courageous step toward reclaiming our lives.

The Foundation of Resilience

Resilience, the ability to bounce back from adversity, is at the heart of conquering depression. It's a trait we can develop and nurture, and it begins with our mindset. We must cultivate a mindset of resilience, one that views setbacks as opportunities for growth rather than insurmountable obstacles. This shift in perspective is the cornerstone of our journey towards healing.

Passion and purpose are not elusive ideals; they're often hidden within us, waiting to be rediscovered. Exploring interests, setting achievable goals, and finding ways to contribute to others' well-being can reignite the spark of purpose. It's a journey of self-discovery and growth, one that can lead individuals out of the depths of depression.

The Power of Positive Self-Talk

Our minds are powerful tools, and they can either uplift us or drag us further into the abyss of depression. Positive self-talk is the key to harnessing this power. Instead of dwelling on negative thoughts and self-criticism, we must consciously replace them with affirmations of self-worth and optimism. By doing so, we rewire our thought patterns, gradually replacing darkness with light.

One of the key components of mindset transformation is learning to reframe negative thoughts. This involves challenging automatic negative thinking and finding more balanced, constructive interpretations of situations. Cognitive Behavioral Therapy (CBT) is a powerful tool in this regard, helping individuals identify and reprogram destructive thought patterns into more positive and constructive thoughts.

Setting Realistic Goals

One of the traps of depression is setting unattainable standards for ourselves. These lofty expectations often lead to disappointment and reinforce feelings of inadequacy. Instead, we should set realistic and achievable goals. These goals, no matter how small they may seem, provide a sense of purpose and accomplishment that is vital in our battle against depression.

Seeking Professional Help

While mindset is a potent tool, it's essential to acknowledge that depression is a complex condition that often requires professional intervention. Seeking help from therapists, counselors, or psychiatrists is a crucial step on our journey to recovery. They provide us with valuable tools and strategies to navigate the labyrinth of depression.

Building a Support Network

No warrior fights alone, and in the battle against depression, a strong support network is invaluable. Surrounding ourselves with understanding friends and family, or connecting with support groups, can provide the emotional bolster we need to face the darkest days.

Building resilience is not a quick fix; it's a journey. It begins with self-awareness, understanding the patterns of thought that contribute to depression. With the help of therapy and support networks, individuals can learn to identify and challenge negative thought patterns, replacing them with healthier alternatives. The journey may also include practices like mindfulness meditation, which can promote emotional regulation and reduce the impact of stressors.

Embracing Self-Care

Self-care is not an indulgence; it's a necessity. Depression often robs us of our vitality, making it all the more important to prioritize self-care. This includes regular exercise, a balanced diet, adequate sleep, and engaging in activities that bring joy. Nurturing our physical and emotional well-being is an integral part of our journey toward light.

Create a personalized self-care routine can provide structure and stability in the face of depression. This routine may include daily exercise, a balanced diet, mindfulness practices, and hobbies that bring joy. Consistency is key, as self-care becomes a lifeline in the journey towards healing.

Resisting Isolation

Depression has a way of isolating us from the world, making us feel alone in our struggle. However, it's crucial to resist this urge to isolate ourselves further. Connecting with others, even when it feels challenging, can provide a lifeline of support and remind us that we are not alone in our battle.

Connecting with others who have experienced or are experiencing depression can be particularly powerful. Support groups and online communities offer a safe space for sharing experiences, gaining insights, and receiving encouragement. These connections can remind individuals that they are not alone in their struggle.

Embracing Mindfulness

Mindfulness practices, such as meditation and deep breathing exercises, can help us gain control over our thoughts and emotions. These practices allow us to stay present in the moment, free from the weight of past regrets or future anxieties. Mindfulness nurtures our mental clarity, leading us closer to the light.

Celebrating Small Victories

As we journey through the abyss of depression, it's essential to celebrate every small victory along the way. Whether it's getting out of bed on a difficult morning or reaching out for help, these victories are not to be underestimated. They are rays of light that pierce through the darkness, reminding us that hope is never truly lost.

The Path to Healing

The power of mindset in battling depression cannot be overstated. It is the compass that guides us from the depths of despair to the heights of resilience. By recognizing the battle within, cultivating resilience, practicing positive self-talk, setting realistic goals, seeking professional help, building a support network, embracing self-care, resisting isolation, adopting mindfulness, and celebrating small victories, we pave the way for our healing journey.

Depression may be a formidable adversary, but with the right mindset, we can transform our lives from darkness to light. Let us remember that, as warriors, we have the power to rewrite our story, one empowered thought at a time.

Chapter 4

Seeking Professional Help: The First Step to Healing from Depression

While it's admirable to want to tackle your problems independently, depression is a formidable opponent. Seeking professional help is a sign of strength, not weakness. It shows that you're willing to do whatever it takes to regain control of your life.

A re you feeling down, overwhelmed, or stuck in a never-ending cycle of sadness? You're not alone. Millions of people around the world grapple with depression every day. It's a silent battle that often goes unnoticed, and it can be incredibly isolating. But here's the good news: there is a way out, and it starts with taking that crucial first step - seeking professional help.

We're going to explore why seeking professional help is your first and most vital step towards healing from depression. We'll dive into the benefits, address common concerns, and provide answers to frequently asked questions. By the end of this journey, you'll not only understand why professional help is essential but also feel empowered to take that step towards a brighter future.

So, let's begin this transformative journey together, with one simple mantra in mind:

Seeking Professional Help: Your First Step to Healing from Depression!

Depression is often misunderstood, and its symptoms can vary widely from person to person. It's not just about feeling sad; it's a complex interplay of emotions, thoughts, and physical sensations that can be incredibly debilitating. Here's a glimpse into the hidden struggles of depression:

The Emotional Rollercoaster

Depression can make you feel like you're riding an emotional rollercoaster with no way off. You might experience:

- Overwhelming sadness
- Irritability
- Hopelessness
- Guilt or shame
- Loss of interest in activities you once enjoyed
- Emotional numbness

The Mental Maze

Depression isn't just about feeling down; it can turn your mind into a labyrinth of negative thoughts and self-doubt:

- Constant self-criticism
- Difficulty concentrating
- Memory problems
- Pervasive negative thinking
- A sense of worthlessness

The Physical Toll

Depression isn't limited to your emotions and thoughts; it can take a toll on your body as well:

- Fatigue and low energy
- Changes in appetite and weight
- Sleep disturbances
- Aches and pains
- Reduced libido

Why "Self-Help" Isn't Always Enough

In the age of the internet, it's tempting to turn to self-help resources when you're dealing with depression. While these resources can be valuable for gaining insights and coping strategies, they often fall short in providing the comprehensive help needed to overcome depression. Here's why:

Lack of Personalization

Depression is highly individualized, and what works for one person may not work for another. Self-help resources provide general advice, but they can't tailor strategies to your unique situation.

Overwhelming Choices

The internet is flooded with self-help articles, books, and videos, making it overwhelming to decide which approach to follow. This can lead to confusion and frustration.

Limited Accountability

When you rely solely on self-help, there's no one holding you accountable for your progress. It's easy to lose motivation and give up when there's no external support system.

The Power of Professional Help

Now that we've explored the challenges of self-help let's delve into the transformative power of seeking professional help:

- *Tailored Treatment Plans-* When you seek professional help, you're not just getting generic advice. You're working with a trained therapist who can create a personalized treatment plan based on your specific needs and goals.

Evidence-Based Approaches- Therapists use evidence-based techniques that have been scientifically proven to help individuals manage and recover from depression. These approaches are rooted in research and have a track record of success.

Support and Accountability- One of the most significant advantages of professional help is the support and accountability it offers. Your therapist becomes your ally in the battle against depression, helping you stay on track and motivated.

Medication Options- In some cases, medication may be a part of your treatment plan. Mental health professionals can assess whether medication is a suitable option for you and monitor its effectiveness.

A Safe Space to Express Yourself- Therapy provides a safe and non-judgmental space where you can express your thoughts and feelings without fear of criticism. It's a place where you're truly heard and understood.

Breaking the Isolation- Depression often makes people feel isolated and disconnected from the world. Therapy can help you reconnect with others, rebuild relationships, and create a support network.

Common Concerns about Seeking Professional Help

Now that you understand the benefits, let's address some common concerns that might be holding you back from taking that crucial step:

"I Can Handle It Myself."

While it's admirable to want to tackle your problems independently, depression is a formidable opponent. Seeking professional help is a sign of strength, not weakness. It shows that you're willing to do whatever it takes to regain control of your life.

"Therapy is Too Expensive."

It's true that therapy can be an investment, but it's an investment in your well-being and future happiness. Many therapists offer sliding scale fees or accept insurance, making it more affordable than you might think. Remember, your mental health is priceless.

"I Don't Want to Be Judged."

Therapists are trained to provide a safe and non-judgmental space for their clients. They're there to support you, not criticize you. Your therapist's primary goal is to help you heal, grow, and thrive.

"What If It Doesn't Work?"

There's no guarantee that any single treatment will work for everyone, but seeking professional help gives you the best chance of success. If one approach doesn't yield the desired results, therapists can adjust your treatment plan or explore alternative strategies.

"I Don't Have Time."

Your mental health should be a priority, and therapy doesn't have to be a time-consuming endeavor. Many therapists offer flexible scheduling, including evening and weekend appointments, to accommodate your busy life.

"I'm Afraid to Open Up."

It's natural to feel apprehensive about opening up to a therapist, especially if you've never been in therapy before. However, therapists are skilled at creating a safe and trusting environment where you can gradually share at your own pace.

Finding the right therapist is essential for a successful therapeutic journey. Here's how you can start your search:

- Ask for recommendations from friends or family.
- Contact your insurance provider for a list of in-network therapists.
- Use online directories or mental health websites to search for therapists in your area.
- Schedule initial consultations with a few therapists to see who you feel most comfortable with.

Your first therapy session is typically an opportunity for you and your therapist to get to know each other. You'll discuss your reasons for seeking therapy and your goals. It's a chance to determine if you and the therapist are a good fit.

The duration of therapy varies from person to person and depends on the severity of your depression and your specific goals. Some individuals may benefit from short-term therapy, while others may engage in longer-term treatment.

Medication is not always necessary for treating depression. It depends on the individual's symptoms and their response to other forms of treatment. Your therapist or psychiatrist will help determine whether medication is appropriate for your situation.

Many therapists offer online therapy sessions, which can be a convenient option for those with busy schedules or limited access to in-person therapy. Online therapy is an effective way to receive support and treatment for depression.

Therapists are bound by ethical guidelines to maintain confidentiality. However, there are legal exceptions to confidentiality in cases where there is a risk of harm to you or others. Your therapist will discuss these limits with you during your initial session.

Depression is a formidable adversary, but it's not one you have to face alone. Seeking professional help is your first step towards healing and reclaiming your life. It's a brave choice that signifies your commitment to your well-being and happiness.

Remember, depression is treatable, and countless individuals have found hope and recovery through therapy and support. It's time to let go of the stigma and misconceptions surrounding mental health treatment and take that leap towards a brighter future.

So, if you've been silently battling depression, it's time to break free from its grip. Seek professional help, and remember, you're not alone on this journey. There is a path to healing, and it begins with you.

Chapter 5

Medication and Therapy: Tools for Recovery from Depression

Recovery from depression is possible, and with the right tools

We'll explore the dynamic duo of medication and therapy and how they can help you or your loved one break free from the clutches of depression.

So, fasten your seatbelts because we're about to embark on a journey through the avenues of recovery, offering you insights, answers, and, most importantly, hope!

Medication: The Silent Supporter

Let's kick things off by talking about the unsung hero in the battle against depression: medication.

How Medication Works

Medication is like that trusty umbrella in a downpour – it won't stop the rain, but it'll keep you dry. In the world of depression, these medications are known as antidepressants, and they work in various ways to alleviate symptoms. Here's the lowdown:

Chemical Balancing Act: Antidepressants help regulate neurotransmitters in your brain, like serotonin and norepinephrine, which play a crucial role in mood regulation. By balancing these chemicals, medication can help improve your overall mood.

Neurogenesis: Some antidepressants stimulate the growth of new brain cells in the hippocampus, a region associated with memory and emotions. This process, known as neurogenesis, can enhance brain function and alleviate depressive symptoms.

Dispelling the Myths

Before you cringe at the idea of medication, let's debunk a few myths that might be swirling in your mind:

Myth #1: Antidepressants are "Happy Pills": Nope, they won't turn you into a perpetual ray of sunshine. Antidepressants aim to bring balance, not unbridled euphoria.

Myth #2: Addiction Risk: Most antidepressants are not addictive. They work differently than drugs that create dependency.

Myth #3: Instant Gratification: Patience is key. Antidepressants may take a few weeks to show their full effects. It's a marathon, not a sprint.

Myth #4: Forever Popping Pills: Antidepressants are not a lifelong commitment for everyone. Your doctor will tailor the treatment plan to your specific needs.

The Right Prescription

Choosing the right medication is like finding the perfect pair of shoes – one size doesn't fit all. It's crucial to work closely with a healthcare professional who can prescribe the most suitable antidepressant for you. Factors like your symptoms, medical history, and potential side effects are all taken into account.

Selective Serotonin Reuptake Inhibitors (SSRIs): These are often the first line of treatment. They include drugs like Prozac, Zoloft, and Lexapro. They increase serotonin levels in the brain.

Serotonin and Norepinephrine Reuptake Inhibitors (SNRIs): Medications like Cymbalta and Effexor target both serotonin and norepinephrine, providing a double punch against depression.

Atypical Antidepressants: When the standard options don't cut it, your doctor may explore atypical antidepressants like *Wellbutrin or Remeron.*

Tricyclic Antidepressants (TCAs): These are older antidepressants that may be used when other options have been exhausted. They have more potential side effects.

Monoamine Oxidase Inhibitors (MAOIs): MAOIs are typically reserved for cases that don't respond to other treatments due to their potential interactions with certain foods and medications.

Side Effects and Managing Them

Like any superhero, even medication has its kryptonite – side effects. But fear not! Most side effects are manageable, and they often diminish as your body adjusts to the medication. Here's a quick rundown of common side effects and how to deal with them:

Nausea: Taking your medication with food can help ease this discomfort.

Insomnia: Your doctor might adjust the timing of your medication or prescribe a sleep aid to combat sleep disturbances.

Sexual Side Effects: It's a real concern for some, but discussing it with your healthcare provider can lead to solutions, like adjusting your medication or adding another to counteract the side effects.

Weight Gain: Regular exercise and a balanced diet can help mitigate this side effect.

Fatigue: This often subsides as your body gets used to the medication. If it persists, your doctor may adjust your dosage.

Combining Medication with Therapy

41

Now that we've explored the world of medication, it's time to introduce its partner in crime – therapy!

Therapy and medication are like peanut butter and jelly – they're fantastic on their own, but when combined, they create something truly special.

Therapy: Unveiling the Power of Talking

Different Flavors of Therapy

Therapy isn't one-size-fits-all either. Just as you have options with medication, you also have various therapeutic approaches to choose from:

Cognitive-Behavioral Therapy (CBT): CBT is like a personal detective for your thoughts. It helps you identify negative thought patterns and replace them with more positive ones.

Psychodynamic Therapy: This type of therapy delves deep into your past experiences and how they might be affecting your present. It's all about uncovering hidden emotions and motives.

Interpersonal Therapy (IPT): IPT focuses on your relationships and how they contribute to your depression. It helps you improve your communication and problem-solving skills.

Mindfulness-Based Cognitive Therapy (MBCT): MBCT combines elements of CBT with mindfulness techniques. It's especially effective in preventing recurrent depression.

Therapy Is Your Safe Space

Therapists are like professional confidants, and your sessions are your judgment-free zone. Here's why therapy can be a game-changer:

Venting Session: Sometimes, all you need is someone to listen – and therapists are excellent listeners!

Tools for Coping: Therapy equips you with an arsenal of coping strategies to deal with life's curveballs.

Unraveling the Knots: It helps you untangle the web of emotions and thoughts that contribute to your depression.

Setting Goals: Therapists help you set realistic goals and track your progress, keeping you on the path to recovery.

The Therapeutic Alliance

Building a strong rapport with your therapist is vital. It's like having a trusty sidekick in your fight against depression. Open communication and trust are the cornerstones of the therapeutic alliance.

Medication vs. Therapy: The Showdown

So, is it medication or therapy? Which one should you choose in your battle against depression? Well, it's not a showdown; it's a partnership!

Here's the deal: medication can help alleviate the most severe symptoms of depression, making it easier for you to engage in therapy effectively. Think of it as medication opening the door to recovery, and therapy guiding you through it.

Finding the Right Balance

The combination of medication and therapy isn't a one-size-fits-all formula. Finding the right balance depends on your unique circumstances. Some may need more emphasis on medication initially, while others may benefit more from therapy. It's all about personalized care.

Tapering Off Medication

The goal is not to be dependent on medication forever. Many individuals can gradually reduce their medication dosage under the supervision of their healthcare provider as their symptoms improve. Therapy then plays a pivotal role in maintaining mental well-being.

You have the freedom to choose, but it's often recommended to explore both avenues for a more comprehensive approach to recovery. Antidepressants can take several weeks to show their full effects, so patience is key.

Some people find relief through lifestyle changes like regular exercise, a balanced diet, and mindfulness practices, but these are often most effective when combined with medication and therapy.

There are low-cost and sliding-scale therapy options available, and some pharmaceutical companies offer assistance programs for medication costs. Don't hesitate to explore these options with your healthcare provider. It's entirely normal to have mixed feelings about seeking help, but remember that depression is an illness, not a personal failing. Seeking help is a sign of strength, not weakness.

In the world of depression, medication and therapy are the dynamic duo you've been waiting for. They are your tools, your allies, and your path to recovery. Whether you choose medication, therapy, or the powerful combination of both, remember this – you're not alone in this journey. Reach out to healthcare professionals, lean on your support system, and never lose hope. Recovery from depression is possible, and with the right tools, you can find your way back to the sunshine, one step at a time.

So, go ahead and take that first step today. Embrace the power of Medication and Therapy: Tools for Recovery from Depression, and let your journey towards a brighter future begin!

Chapter 6

Building a Strong Support System to Overcome Depression

Depression can be isolating, making you believe that you're alone in your suffering. However, as Many have walked this path before you and have emerged stronger, wiser, and whole again. You can too.

Do you ever find yourself feeling trapped in the murky depths of depression, struggling to find a way out? You're not alone in this battle. Depression can be a relentless foe, but it's a fight you can win, especially when you have a strong support system by your side. We will delve into the importance of building a robust support network to overcome depression, offering insights, tips, and real-life stories that will inspire you on your journey towards recovery.

Depression is a challenging adversary, but it's crucial to remember that you don't have to face it alone. With the right support system in place, you can regain control of your life and rediscover the joy and purpose that depression may have stolen from you. Let's embark on this journey together and explore how to build a strong support system that can help you conquer depression once and for all.

The Power of Connection: Why a Support System Matters

Depression often thrives in isolation, convincing you that you're alone in your struggles. However, one of the most potent weapons against depression is the support of others.

Here's why having a strong support system is vital in the battle against depression:

Emotional Resilience: Depression can be emotionally draining, making it challenging to cope with daily life. A support system provides you with a safety net of emotional support, allowing you to bounce back from the darkest moments.

Perspective and Validation: Depression can distort your perception of reality, making you feel as though there's no way out. Trusted friends and family can offer an objective perspective, helping you see that your thoughts and feelings are not all-encompassing truths.

Practical Assistance: Sometimes, the most basic tasks can seem insurmountable when you're depressed. A strong support system can step in to help with daily chores, errands, or simply lending a listening ear.

Reduced Stigma: Sharing your struggles with a support system can help break the stigma surrounding depression. The more we open up about mental health, the easier it becomes for others to seek help as well.

Who Can Be Part of Your Support System?

Now that we understand why a support system is essential, let's explore who can be part of it:

Family: Your family members, such as parents, siblings, or children, often form the foundation of your support system. They have a deep understanding of your history and can provide unwavering love and care.

Friends: Close friends who have been with you through thick and thin can be invaluable. They offer companionship, a shoulder to cry on, and the occasional distraction that can brighten your day.

Mental Health Professionals: Therapists, counselors, and psychiatrists are trained to help individuals cope with depression. Their expertise can provide you with tailored strategies and treatment options.

Support Groups: Joining a support group for depression can connect you with people who share similar experiences. Sharing and listening to others' stories can be incredibly therapeutic.

Pets: The unconditional love of a furry friend can provide comfort during challenging times. Pets offer companionship and a reason to get out of bed on difficult days.

Online Communities: In today's digital age, you can find support and understanding online. Various forums, chat groups, and social media platforms have communities dedicated to mental health.

Workplace Support: Some workplaces offer Employee Assistance Programs (EAPs) that provide counseling and support for employees facing mental health challenges. Human resources or a trusted colleague can guide you to these resources.

Remember that your support system doesn't have to be extensive. Quality matters more than quantity. Even one or two people who genuinely care about your well-being can make a world of difference.

Building Your Support System: Practical Steps

Now that we've identified who can be part of your support system, let's dive into the steps for building it:

1. Open Up About Your Depression

Breaking the silence is the first crucial step. Let your trusted individuals know what you're going through. Sharing your feelings, thoughts, and experiences can be difficult, but it's essential for them to understand your journey.

2. Seek Professional Help

A mental health professional should be a cornerstone of your support system. They can provide you with a diagnosis, treatment options, and coping strategies tailored to your specific needs. Don't hesitate to reach out to a therapist or psychiatrist for guidance.

3. Set Realistic Expectations

Recovery from depression is not a linear path, and setbacks are normal. Be patient with yourself and your support system. Understanding that there will be good and bad days can help manage expectations.

4. Communicate Your Needs

Your support system is not mind readers. If you need someone to talk to, assistance with daily tasks, or simply some company, express your needs clearly. Effective communication ensures that your support system can provide the help you require.

5. Establish Boundaries

While your support system is essential, it's also crucial to maintain boundaries. Don't rely on them too heavily, and be considerate of their own needs and limitations. Balance is key to healthy relationships within your support network.

6. Join Support Groups

Consider joining a local or online support group for individuals with depression. These groups provide a sense of belonging and understanding that can be incredibly comforting.

7. Self-Care

Self-care is not selfish; it's a necessity. Make sure to prioritize self-care activities that nurture your mental and emotional well-being. This might include exercise, meditation, or pursuing hobbies you enjoy.

8. Be a Supportive Friend

Remember that relationships are a two-way street. Just as you receive support, be prepared to offer it to others in your support network when they need it. Building a reciprocal system fosters trust and mutual care.

9. Regularly Evaluate Your Support System

As time passes, the composition of your support system may change. People may come and go, and that's okay. Periodically assess your support network to ensure it aligns with your current needs and goals.

Real-Life Stories: Triumph over Depression

To illustrate the power of a strong support system, let's explore a few real-life stories of individuals who successfully overcame depression with the help of their networks.

Sarah's Journey

Sarah, a young woman in her twenties, battled depression for several years in silence. She was afraid to burden her family and friends with her struggles until one day, she confided in her childhood friend, Emma. Emma became Sarah's anchor, encouraging her to seek professional help. With therapy and medication, Sarah began her journey to recovery. Along the way, she also joined an online support group, where she found understanding and shared experiences. Today, Sarah is thriving, and her bond with Emma remains unbreakable.

Jason's Transformation

Jason, a middle-aged man, had been dealing with depression for most of his adult life. He felt isolated and didn't want to burden his family, who were unaware of his struggles. It wasn't until he opened up to a therapist that he began to see a glimmer of hope. His therapist encouraged him to reconnect with his estranged son, James, who had moved abroad. Over time, their relationship blossomed, and James became an integral part of Jason's support system. Together, they worked through the challenges of depression, proving that even fractured relationships can heal.

While mental health professionals are essential, a comprehensive support system often includes friends and family who offer emotional support and a sense of belonging. It's a combination of professional guidance and personal connections that can make a significant difference in your journey to recovery.

It can be challenging when loved ones don't understand depression. Consider sharing educational resources with them or attending therapy sessions together to foster understanding. If they remain unsupportive, lean on friends, support groups, or online communities for additional support.

To find a suitable therapist or counselor, start by researching licensed mental health professionals in your area or those available through teletherapy. You can also ask for recommendations from your primary care physician or use online directories provided by mental health organizations.

Quality of friends matters more than quantity when it comes to support systems. Focus on building deeper connections with the people you trust, and consider joining support groups or seeking online communities where you can connect with like-minded individuals.

Medication can be a valuable component of treatment for many individuals with depression. It's essential to consult with a mental health professional who can assess your specific needs and discuss the potential benefits and side effects of medication.

It's time to reassess your support system if you notice changes in your relationships, your needs have evolved, or if you feel that certain individuals are no longer providing the support you require. Regular self-reflection can help you determine when adjustments are needed.

Building a strong support system to overcome depression is not a sign of weakness; it's a testament to your strength and resilience. Depression is a formidable opponent, but with the right network of friends, family, professionals, and even pets, you can face it head-on and emerge victorious.

Remember that your journey to recovery may have its ups and downs, but that's perfectly normal. By opening up about your depression, seeking professional help, and nurturing your support network, you can regain control of your life. Real-life stories like Sarah's and Mike's serve as a testament to the transformative power of human connection and support.

So, don't hesitate to reach out, share your struggles, and start building your own strong support system today. Together, you can overcome depression and rediscover the beauty and joy that life has to offer. Building a strong support system to overcome depression is not just an option; it's a lifeline to a brighter future.

Chapter 7

Harnessing the Healing Power of Self-Care to Overcome Depression

Self-care encompasses activities that promote relaxation, rejuvenation, and overall health.

Depression can feel like an endless storm cloud hovering over your life, casting shadows on your thoughts and emotions. It's an insidious adversary that affects millions worldwide. However, there's a ray of hope that shines through the gloom

So, you might be wondering: What is self-care, and how can it truly help overcome depression? Well, grab a cozy blanket and a warm cup of tea because we're about to embark on a journey that delves deep into the world of self-care, exploring its profound effects on mental health. Let's get started!

The Self-Care Revolution

When you hear the term "self-care," you might envision bubble baths and scented candles – and you're not entirely wrong! But self-care is far more than that. It's a comprehensive approach to nurturing your physical, emotional, and mental well-being.

Self-care encompasses activities that promote relaxation, rejuvenation, and overall health.

It involves listening to your body, recognizing your needs, and taking deliberate actions to fulfill them.

Self-care is a powerful tool for managing stress, improving mood, and combating depression.

The Science behind Self-Care

Now, you might be thinking, "Okay, that all sounds nice, but is there any science behind it?" Absolutely! The science of self-care is grounded in the intricate relationship between body and mind.

When you engage in self-care activities, your brain releases endorphins – those feel-good chemicals that act as natural mood lifters.

Studies have shown that self-care can reduce the production of stress hormones like cortisol, which are often elevated in individuals with depression.

Additionally, practicing self-care can enhance the brain's neuroplasticity, making it more resilient to depressive symptoms.

So, in essence, self-care isn't just a trendy buzzword; it's a scientifically proven method for improving mental health.

The Depression Dilemma

Depression isn't merely feeling a little down or having a bad day. It's a persistent, complex, and often debilitating mental health condition that affects every facet of life.

People with depression may experience overwhelming sadness, hopelessness, and a loss of interest in once-enjoyable activities.

Fatigue, changes in appetite, sleep disturbances, and difficulty concentrating are common symptoms.

Depression can lead to a sense of isolation, strained relationships, and even physical health problems.

Navigating the labyrinth of depression can be incredibly challenging, but self-care offers a glimmer of hope in the darkest of times.

Self-Care Strategies for Depression

Let's dive headfirst into the heart of the matter – how can you harness the healing power of self-care to overcome depression? Here are some tried-and-true strategies:

1. Prioritize Sleep

Sleep is your body's reset button. Without adequate rest, your mental health can take a nosedive. Try these tips:

Establish a consistent sleep schedule.

Create a calming bedtime routine and limit screen time before bed.

2. Move Your Body

Exercise isn't just for physical health; it's a potent ally in the battle against depression. You can engage in activities you enjoy, whether it's dancing, hiking, or yoga. Exercise releases endorphins and can improve self-esteem.

3. Nourish Your Body

A well-balanced diet can have a profound impact on your mood and energy levels. Focus on whole foods rich in nutrients. Always stay hydrated – even mild dehydration can affect your mood.

4. Embrace Mindfulness

Mindfulness practices can help you stay grounded and reduce the impact of depressive thoughts. Try meditation, deep breathing exercises, or progressive muscle relaxation. Stay present in the moment, rather than dwelling on the past or worrying about the future.

5. Seek Support

Don't go it alone – reach out to friends, family, or a therapist. Sharing your feelings can provide relief and connection. Professional guidance can help you develop coping strategies.

6. Engage in Creative Outlets

Expressing yourself through art, writing, or any creative outlet can be incredibly therapeutic. Creative activities can serve as a release for pent-up emotions. They offer a sense of accomplishment and self-expression.

7. Set Realistic Goals

Depression can make even the simplest tasks feel daunting. Break them down into manageable steps. Celebrate small victories. Avoid overwhelming yourself with unrealistic expectations.

8. Establish Boundaries

Don't spread yourself too thin – learn to say no when necessary. Setting boundaries protects your mental and emotional well-being. It's okay to put yourself first sometimes.

Expert Insights: The Therapist's Perspective

We've explored some practical self-care strategies, but it's crucial to understand how therapists view the role of self-care in overcoming depression. To gain further insight, we spoke to Dr. Sarah Anderson, a licensed therapist with over a decade of experience.

Dr. Anderson's Take on Self-Care

Dr. Anderson emphasizes that self-care is a vital component of managing depression:

"It's not selfish; it's self-preservation. I often encourage my clients to view self-care as a non-negotiable part of their routine. Just like you wouldn't skip brushing your teeth, you shouldn't skip self-care activities that promote your mental health."

She also stresses the importance of customization:

"Self-care isn't one-size-fits-all. It's about finding what works for you personally. Some people find solace in nature, while others prefer creative outlets. The key is to experiment and discover what resonates with you."

Personal Stories: Triumph through Self-Care

To truly appreciate the transformative potential of self-care, let's hear from individuals who have battled depression and emerged stronger, thanks to their self-care journeys.

Jane's Journey: Finding Serenity in Nature

Jane, a 34-year-old artist, struggled with depression for years. She describes how nature became her refuge:

"Whenever I felt the weight of depression, I'd head to the nearby park. The simple act of being in nature, surrounded by trees and birdsong, felt like a healing balm for my soul. It gave me a break from the constant turmoil in my mind."

Jane's story highlights the therapeutic power of connecting with the natural world as a form of self-care.

Mike's Odyssey: The Healing Magic of Music

Mike, a 42-year-old musician, battled depression throughout his career. He shares his transformative experience:

"Music has always been my sanctuary. When I was at my lowest, I started composing music that expressed my emotions. It was like pouring my heart out without words. Music became my lifeline, and it still is."

Mike's story underscores how creative outlets can be powerful tools for self-expression and healing.

Can self-care completely cure depression?

Self-care is a valuable tool for managing depression and improving overall well-being. However, it may not be a standalone cure for severe depression. In such cases, professional help, including therapy and medication, may be necessary.

Experimentation is key to finding the right self-care activities for you. Try various self-care activities to see what resonates with you. It could be anything from reading a book to going for a run. Listen to your body and mind to discover what brings you peace and joy.

Self-care is an act of self-compassion. It allows you to recharge, so you can better support yourself and others. It's about preserving your mental and emotional health, which ultimately benefits everyone around you.

In fact, incorporating self-care into your daily routine can be highly effective. Start with small steps, such as setting aside time for meditation or a brief walk, and gradually expand your self-care practices.

Prioritizing self-care can be challenging, especially when depression looms. Consider enlisting the support of a therapist or a trusted friend who can help you establish a self-care routine and hold you accountable.

So, whether you find solace in the simplicity of a daily walk in the park, the soothing rhythm of your favorite song, or the cathartic release of creative expression, know that self-care is a beacon of hope on your path to healing.

Incorporate self-care into your daily life, seek support when needed, and remember that you are not alone in your battle against depression. Together with the therapeutic insights of professionals and the inspiring stories of individuals who have triumphed, you can unlock the transformative potential of self-care, casting aside the shadows of depression and embracing a brighter, more fulfilling future.

Chapter 8

Unmasking the Stigma of Depression

The brightest smiles hide the deepest pain

Depression is a topic that's been shrouded in secrecy for far too long? Welcome to a candid conversation about depression, that elusive shadow that affects millions of lives worldwide. We're going to tear down the curtains of stigma and reveal the raw, unfiltered truth about depression. Get ready to explore the depths of this often-misunderstood mental health condition, as we aim to demystify, destigmatize, and ultimately provide support and understanding.

So, what's the deal with depression? Why do so many suffer in silence, and how can we help? Let's start the journey together as we unmask the stigma of depression and shed light on the path to healing.

Unmasking the Myths

Myth 1: "Depression is Just a Bad Mood, Right?"

Let's kick things off by debunking one of the most common misconceptions about depression. No, it's not just a "bad mood" that you can shake off with a cup of coffee and a cheerful playlist. Depression is a complex mental health disorder with a wide range of symptoms, including:

- Persistent sadness
- Loss of interest in once-enjoyed activities
- Fatigue
- Changes in appetite or weight
- Sleep disturbances
- Feelings of worthlessness or guilt
- Difficulty concentrating
- Thoughts of death or suicide

These symptoms can persist for weeks, months, or even years, significantly impacting a person's quality of life. Depression is not a fleeting emotion; it's a serious medical condition that requires attention and care.

Myth 2: "People with Depression are Just Lazy or Weak"

Another harmful myth that needs to be unmasked is the idea that people with depression are simply lazy or weak-willed. In reality, depression is a biological, psychological, and social condition that can affect anyone, regardless of their strength or willpower. Factors such as genetics, brain chemistry, and life experiences all play a role in the development of depression.

Imagine carrying an invisible weight that makes every step feel like a marathon, every task seem insurmountable, and every decision an agonizing choice. That's what living with depression can feel like. It takes immense strength to face each day when your own mind seems to be working against you.

The Hidden Struggles

One of the most insidious aspects of depression is the isolation it breeds. When someone is struggling with depression, they often feel like they're alone in their battle. This sense of isolation can be compounded by the fear of judgment and stigma from others. It's a cruel cycle that keeps many from seeking help.

Why do people with depression isolate themselves?

Isolation can be a coping mechanism for those with depression. They might withdraw from social interactions because they feel like a burden to others or because they're too exhausted to engage. It's crucial to understand that this withdrawal isn't a choice but a symptom of the condition.

The Smile That Hides the Pain

Ever heard the phrase, "The brightest smiles hide the deepest pain"? Well, it couldn't be truer when it comes to depression. Many individuals with depression become experts at wearing a mask, concealing their true emotions behind a façade of happiness. They don't want to burden others with their struggles, so they put on a brave face even when they're crumbling inside.

Why do people with depression hide their feelings?

The fear of being judged or misunderstood often drives people with depression to hide their feelings. They worry that opening up about their pain will make others uncomfortable or lead to rejection. It's essential to create a safe and non-judgmental environment for them to share their emotions.

Breaking the Chains of Stigma

The first step in unmasking the stigma of depression is to start talking about it openly and honestly. When we bring the topic out of the shadows, we create a space where those affected can feel safe and understood.

How can I start a conversation about depression with someone I care about?

Approach the conversation with empathy and care. Let them know you're there to listen without judgment. Use open-ended questions to encourage them to share their feelings, and validate their experiences by expressing your concern and support.

Educating Ourselves

Knowledge is power, and when it comes to depression, understanding is key. Take the time to educate yourself about depression, its symptoms, and its treatment options. The more informed you are, the better equipped you are to support your loved ones.

Where can I find reliable information about depression?

You can start by exploring reputable websites like the National Institute of Mental Health (NIMH) or consulting with mental health professionals. Books and documentaries about depression can also provide valuable insights.

Dismantling Stereotypes

It's time to challenge the stereotypes and misconceptions that surround depression. No, depression is not a sign of weakness, and it's certainly not something that can be wished away. By confronting these stereotypes, we can create a more empathetic and inclusive society.

How can I help combat stereotypes about depression?

Speak up when you encounter stereotypes or stigmatizing language. Share your knowledge about depression to help dispel myths. Encourage open conversations about mental health in your community and workplace.

A Beacon of Hope

Depression is treatable, and seeking help is a sign of strength, not weakness. If you or someone you know is struggling with depression, it's essential to reach out for support.

Who can I turn to for help with depression?

Mental health professionals: Therapists, counselors, and psychiatrists can provide therapy and medication options.

Support groups: Joining a support group can connect you with others who understand your struggles.

Friends and family: Lean on your loved ones for emotional support.

The Role of Therapy

Therapy is a valuable tool in the journey to recovery from depression. It provides a safe and confidential space to explore your thoughts and feelings, learn coping strategies, and work towards healing.

What types of therapy are effective for depression?

Several types of therapy can be beneficial for depression, including:

- Cognitive-behavioral therapy (CBT)
- Interpersonal therapy (IPT)
- Dialectical behavior therapy (DBT)
- Mindfulness-based cognitive therapy (MBCT)
- Medication as a Treatment Option

In some cases, medication may be prescribed to help manage the symptoms of depression. Antidepressants can be a useful part of a treatment plan, but they should always be used under the guidance of a medical professional.

Are antidepressants safe, and do they have side effects?

Antidepressants are generally safe when prescribed and monitored by a healthcare provider. Like any medication, they can have side effects, but these are typically mild and temporary. It's essential to discuss any concerns or side effects with your healthcare provider.

Depression is a complex and challenging condition, but it's one that can be understood and managed with the right support.

Remember, depression is not a sign of weakness, and seeking help is an act of courage. By opening up conversations, challenging stereotypes, and providing support, we can create a world where those affected by depression no longer need to hide behind a mask of smiles. Let's continue to unmask the stigma and offer compassion, understanding, and hope to all those who need it.

So, the next time you encounter someone struggling with depression, be the beacon of light that helps them unmask their pain and find the path to healing. Together, we can make a difference in the lives of those who need it most.

Chapter 9

Finding Hope in Daily Practices

Even the steepest mountains can be conquered, and the journey itself can become rewarding

D epression is like a persistent raincloud that refuses to budge. It can cast a shadow over even the sunniest days, making life seem gray and unbearable. But, my friend, there's hope! There are daily practices that can help you find that glimmer of hope even on your darkest days. We're not talking about quick fixes or miracle cures; we're talking about the small, manageable steps you can take to gradually improve your mental health. So, let's embark on this journey of Finding Hope in Daily Practices when dealing with depression!

The Battle with Depression: A Daily Struggle

Living with depression can feel like trying to climb a mountain with a backpack full of rocks. Each step is heavy, and the destination often seems distant and unreachable. But, remember, even the steepest mountains can be conquered, and the journey itself can become rewarding. Here are some daily practices that can help you in your battle with depression.

1. Morning Rituals: Setting the Tone for the Day

Start with Gratitude

The moment you open your eyes, take a deep breath, and think about the things you're grateful for. It could be as simple as the warm embrace of your blanket or the aroma of fresh coffee brewing in the kitchen. Starting your day with gratitude can help shift your focus away from negative thoughts.

Mindful Breathing

Before you jump out of bed, spend a few minutes practicing mindful breathing. Inhale slowly and deeply, counting to four, then exhale, counting to four again. This simple exercise can calm your mind and reduce anxiety, making it easier to face the day.

Set Small Goals

Don't overwhelm yourself with a long to-do list. Instead, set small, achievable goals for the day. Whether it's making your bed, going for a short walk, or completing a work task, accomplishing these goals can give you a sense of purpose and accomplishment.

2. Nourish Your Body and Mind

Balanced Diet

Your body and mind are closely connected, and what you eat can impact your mood. Aim for a balanced diet rich in fruits, vegetables, whole grains, and lean proteins. Avoid excessive caffeine and sugar, as they can lead to energy crashes and mood swings.

Stay Hydrated

Dehydration can exacerbate feelings of fatigue and irritability. Make sure you're drinking enough water throughout the day. Try carrying a reusable water bottle with you as a reminder.

Mindful Eating

Eating mindfully means savoring each bite, paying attention to the flavors and textures. It's not just about what you eat but how you eat it. This practice can help you develop a healthier relationship with food and reduce emotional eating.

3. The Power of Connection

Reach Out to Loved Ones

Isolation can be a breeding ground for depression. Force yourself, if necessary, to reach out to friends and family. Even a brief conversation or a text message exchange can remind you that you're not alone.

Join Support Groups

Consider joining a local or online support group for people dealing with depression. Sharing your experiences with others who understand can provide a sense of belonging and support.

4. Embrace Physical Activity

Start Slow

Exercise releases endorphins, the body's natural mood elevators. However, if the thought of hitting the gym is overwhelming, start slow. Take short walks, practice gentle yoga, or dance in your living room. The key is to move your body regularly.

Outdoor Adventures

Getting some fresh air and sunlight can do wonders for your mood. Go for a hike, have a picnic in the park, or simply sit in your backyard and soak up the sun.

Find an Exercise Buddy

Sometimes, having a workout partner can be incredibly motivating. Convince a friend or family member to join you on your fitness journey.

5. Mindfulness and Meditation

Daily Meditation

Take a few minutes each day to meditate. Find a quiet space, sit comfortably, and focus on your breath. Let go of intrusive thoughts and just be in the moment.

Mindful Awareness

Practice mindfulness throughout the day. Pay attention to your thoughts and feelings without judgment. This can help you gain control over negative thought patterns.

6. Creativity and Expression

Creative Outlets

Engaging in creative activities can be therapeutic. Whether it's painting, writing, playing an instrument, or gardening, find something that allows you to express yourself.

Journaling

Keeping a journal can help you process your emotions and track your progress. Write down your thoughts and feelings, and look back to see how far you've come.

7. Sleep Hygiene

Establish a Routine

Create a bedtime routine that signals to your body that it's time to wind down. Avoid screens before bedtime, keep your bedroom dark and cool, and try relaxation techniques such as deep breathing or progressive muscle relaxation.

Consistent Sleep Schedule

Try to go to bed and wake up at the same time every day, even on weekends. Consistency can improve the quality of your sleep.

Can these daily practices really help with depression?

Absolutely! While they may not provide an instant cure, these daily practices can gradually improve your mental health and help you manage depression better.

What if I don't have the energy to do any of these activities?

Start small and be patient with yourself. Even the tiniest steps can make a difference. Over time, you'll find that your energy and motivation improve.

Should I seek professional help alongside these practices?

If your depression is severe or persistent, it's essential to seek professional help. These practices can complement therapy and medication but should not replace them if they are medically necessary.

Depression is undoubtedly a formidable opponent, but with daily practices, you can regain a sense of control and find hope in each passing day. Remember, it's okay to have setbacks and difficult moments, but these practices can be your lifeline during those times.

So, start your day with gratitude, nourish your body and mind, reach out to loved ones, embrace physical activity, practice mindfulness, and let your creativity shine. With consistent effort and self-compassion, you can find hope in daily practices when dealing with depression. The journey won't always be easy, but the rewards are worth it. You've got this!

Incorporate these practices into your daily routine, and you'll slowly but surely see that persistent raincloud begin to dissipate, allowing the sun to break through, warming your heart and lighting your path towards a brighter future.

Chapter 10

Navigating the Rollercoaster of Emotions

Learn to embrace the small victories, no matter how insignificant they may seem.

Depression, often misunderstood and stigmatized, is not just a singular state of mind. It's a multifaceted experience that can leave you feeling like you're on an emotional rollercoaster.

It comes with highs and lows, twists and turns, and unexpected loops. From the depths of despair to moments of surprising clarity, we'll delve into the complexities of this mental health challenge. Whether you're someone living with depression or seeking to understand a loved one's experience, we've got you covered.

So, grab your emotional safety harness and let's navigate the rollercoaster of emotions that is depression together!

The Loop of Denial

When depression first creeps into your life, it often begins with a subtle, creeping darkness that clouds your thoughts. You might find yourself experiencing inexplicable sadness, lack of motivation, or persistent fatigue. At this stage, it's easy to deny that anything is wrong. "It's just a phase," you might tell yourself. "I'll snap out of it."

But beware! Denial is the first loop on this rollercoaster, and it's a steep one. The more you deny the existence of depression, the faster and deeper you plunge into its grip.

Sharp Turns of Self-Doubt

As the rollercoaster descends, you'll encounter sharp turns of self-doubt. You may question your worth, your abilities, and even your purpose in life. This is where depression gets cunning, convincing you that these negative thoughts are your new reality. You might start isolating yourself, avoiding social interactions, and withdrawing from activities you once loved.

Tip: If you suspect depression, don't ignore it. Seek support from friends, family, or a mental health professional. Early intervention can prevent the rollercoaster from spiraling out of control!

The Ups and Downs of Coping

Just when you think you've hit rock bottom, depression throws you a curveball. It's called "The False Peaks of Temporary Relief." Suddenly, you feel a bit better. You may have a good day or even a great week. It's during these moments that you convince yourself, "I'm cured!"

But hold on tight! This is one of the trickiest parts of the rollercoaster. The relief is often temporary, and you can quickly find yourself plummeting back into the depths of despair.

The Twisted Tunnel of Self-Medication

When the rollercoaster takes a nosedive, you might seek ways to numb the pain. This is where the Twisted Tunnel of Self-Medication comes into play. Some people turn to alcohol, drugs, or other unhealthy coping mechanisms in an attempt to escape the relentless grip of depression.

Remember: Self-medication is a loop within a loop, a dangerous cycle that only intensifies the rollercoaster ride. Seek healthier ways to cope, such as therapy, exercise, or creative outlets.

The Loop of Acceptance

After several spins on the rollercoaster, you might reach a point where you can't deny depression any longer. This is the beginning of the Loop of Acceptance. It's not an easy climb, but it's a crucial one.

As you accept your condition, you open the door to healing. You might start therapy or medication, and you'll likely find solace in sharing your struggles with others who understand.

How can you start the climb towards acceptance?

Reach out to a therapist, counselor, or support group. Acceptance is the first step towards a smoother ride.

The Serpentine Path of Recovery

The Loop of Acceptance leads you to the Serpentine Path of Recovery. It's a winding, unpredictable journey filled with moments of progress and setbacks. Just like a rollercoaster, recovery has its ups and downs.

During recovery, you'll discover newfound strength and resilience within yourself. You'll also learn to embrace the small victories, no matter how insignificant they may seem.

The Loop of Relapse

Recovery isn't always a one-way ticket to emotional stability. Depression can throw you for a loop with the unexpected and disheartening plunge of relapse. You might have been feeling better, but suddenly, you're back in the depths of despair. This can be discouraging and disorienting.

But remember: Relapse is a common part of the journey, not a sign of failure. It's okay to seek help and support when you experience a relapse.

The Bumpy Road of Resilience

The Loop of Relapse isn't just about the fall; it's also about how you bounce back. The road to resilience can be bumpy and filled with challenges, but it's a vital part of the rollercoaster ride.

Resilience means learning from setbacks, adjusting your coping strategies, and continuing to move forward. It's the determination to keep riding the rollercoaster, even when it feels like it's trying to throw you off.

Is relapse a sign that I'm not getting better?

Not at all. Relapse is a common part of the recovery process. It's a detour, not a dead-end.

How can I cope with a relapse?

Reach out to your support system, whether it's friends, family, or a therapist. Don't go through it alone.

Will I ever fully recover from depression?

Full recovery is possible, but it's different for everyone. The rollercoaster may never disappear completely, but its twists and turns can become more manageable.

The Loop of Resilience

As you continue to navigate the rollercoaster, you'll experience the thrill of resilience. This is the loop where you realize just how far you've come. You'll recognize the inner strength and determination that have carried you through the toughest twists and turns.

Embrace the thrill! Celebrate your victories, no matter how small they may seem. They are proof of your resilience.

The Smooth Ride of Self-Care

The Loop of Resilience leads to the Smooth Ride of Self-Care. At this point, you've learned the importance of taking care of your mental health. Self-care becomes a non-negotiable part of your life.

Self-care isn't just about bubble baths and spa days (although those can be nice!). It's about setting boundaries, practicing mindfulness, and prioritizing your well-being.

Pro tip: Make a self-care plan that includes activities you genuinely enjoy. It'll make the rollercoaster ride more bearable.

The Loop of Empathy

One unexpected twist of the rollercoaster is the Loop of Empathy. Through your own struggles, you become more compassionate and understanding towards others. You can relate to their emotional ups and downs in a way you couldn't before.

Empathy allows you to be a source of support for friends and loved ones who may be facing their own battles with depression. You're not just riding the rollercoaster for yourself; you're in it together with others.

How can you show empathy towards someone struggling with depression?

Listen without judgment, offer a shoulder to lean on, and let them know they're not alone in this emotional rollercoaster.

The Loop of Advocacy

The Loop of Empathy often leads to the Loop of Advocacy. When you've experienced the rollercoaster of depression, you're more likely to advocate for mental health awareness and support.

You might share your story, participate in mental health initiatives, or become a champion for accessible mental health care. Your journey becomes a source of inspiration for others.

How can I start advocating for mental health?

Start by sharing your story with friends and family. You can also get involved in local or online mental health organizations.

Is it okay to be open about my own struggles?

Absolutely! Sharing your experiences can help reduce stigma and encourage others to seek help.

In the world of depression, navigating the rollercoaster of emotions is a challenging and unpredictable journey. It's a ride filled with loops of denial, coping, acceptance, relapse, resilience, empathy, and advocacy. Each loop presents its own set of challenges and triumphs, making the rollercoaster experience unique for every individual.

Remember, you're not alone on this rollercoaster. Reach out to your support system, seek professional help when needed, and practice self-care along the way. Embrace the loops of empathy and advocacy, knowing that your journey can inspire and support others.

So, as you continue riding the rollercoaster of emotions that is depression, hold on tight, stay resilient, and know that brighter days are ahead. The loops may be daunting, but they are also a testament to your strength and courage. Keep on navigating, and you'll find your way to a smoother ride.

Embrace the rollercoaster, for it is a part of your story, and it is a story worth telling!

Chapter 11

Understanding Mindfulness and Meditation for Managing Depression

When you're mindful, you're not dwelling on the past or stressing about the future

I n a world that often feels like a non-stop rollercoaster ride, it's not uncommon for many of us to experience moments of depression and anxiety. The fast-paced nature of our lives, coupled with the pressures of work, relationships, and personal expectations, can weigh us down. But what if there was a way to find calm amidst the chaos, a respite for your mind? Enter the powerful duo of mindfulness and meditation, a dynamic duo that can play a significant role in managing depression.

What is Mindfulness?

To kick things off, let's clarify what mindfulness is all about. Essentially, mindfulness is the practice of being present, fully engaged in the here and now. It's about tuning into your thoughts, feelings, and bodily sensations without judgment. Sounds easy, right? Well, in our age of constant distractions, it can be a real challenge!

A Moment's Peace: How Mindfulness Works

So, how does mindfulness help in managing depression? It's all about giving your mind a breather. When you're mindful, you're not dwelling on the past or stressing about the future. Instead, you're focusing on the present moment, allowing yourself to experience it without the weight of negative thoughts dragging you down.

The Science behind It: Mindfulness and Depression

You might wonder, is there any science to back this up? Absolutely! Researchers have found that practicing mindfulness can lead to reduced symptoms of depression. This is because it helps break the cycle of rumination and negative thinking, which are common culprits in fueling depression.

What is Meditation?

Meditation is like a mental gym for your brain. It involves focusing your mind on a particular object, thought, or activity to train your attention and awareness.

How Meditation Works

Imagine your mind as a turbulent sea during a storm. Meditation is the anchor that helps you find calm amidst the chaos. By practicing meditation regularly, you can develop greater control over your thoughts and emotions, which is particularly valuable when dealing with depression.

The Brain's Best Friend: Meditation and Depression

What's the connection between meditation and depression? Well, studies have shown that meditation can lead to increased levels of *serotonin* and *dopamine*, the brain's feel-good chemicals. It's like a natural antidepressant, but without any side effects!

Mindfulness and Meditation: How They Complement Each Other

Think of mindfulness as the foundation, the practice that helps you become aware of your thoughts and feelings. Meditation, on the other hand, is the tool that allows you to control and redirect those thoughts and feelings in a positive direction.

The Power of the Present: How They Tackle Depression

Imagine this scenario: you're feeling overwhelmed by negative thoughts and emotions. Your mind is like a wild horse, uncontrollable and racing in all directions. This is where mindfulness steps in. It helps you rein in that wild horse, bringing you back to the present moment. You acknowledge those negative thoughts and feelings without judgment.

Now, here's where meditation enters the picture. Once you're grounded in the present, meditation provides you with the tools to reshape those negative thoughts. It's like sculpting your mental landscape, molding it into a place of positivity and tranquility. This powerful combination can be a game-changer in managing depression.

Putting It into Practice: Mindfulness and Meditation Techniques

Mindful Breathing

One of the simplest ways to practice mindfulness is through mindful breathing. Here's how to do it:

- Find a quiet place where you won't be disturbed.
- Sit or lie down comfortably.
- Close your eyes.
- Take a deep breath in through your nose, counting to four.
- Exhale slowly through your mouth, counting to six.
- Repeat this process, focusing your attention solely on your breath.

Whenever your mind starts to wander (and it will), gently bring your focus back to your breath. This exercise can be incredibly effective in reducing stress and promoting relaxation.

Dive Deeper: Body Scan Meditation

Body scan meditation is a wonderful way to connect with your body and release tension. Here's how it works:

- Find a comfortable and quiet place to sit or lie down.
- Close your eyes.
- Begin by focusing your attention on your toes. Pay close attention to any sensations or tension you may feel in this area.
- Slowly move your attention up through your body, from your toes to your head, noticing any areas of tension or discomfort.
- Breathe deeply and imagine each breath melting away the tension in each part of your body.

This practice can help you become more aware of physical sensations and relax your body, which can, in turn, ease your mind.

Common Questions about Mindfulness and Meditation for Depression

1. Can mindfulness and meditation cure depression?

While they are powerful tools, mindfulness and meditation are not a cure for depression. They are best used as part of a holistic approach to managing depression, which may include therapy, medication, and lifestyle changes.

2. How long does it take to see results from mindfulness and meditation?

The timeline for experiencing the benefits of mindfulness and meditation can vary from person to person. Some people may notice improvements in their mood and well-being within a few weeks of regular practice, while others may take longer. Consistency is key, so keep at it!

3. Can anyone practice mindfulness and meditation?

Yes, absolutely! Mindfulness and meditation are practices that can be adapted to suit individuals of all ages and backgrounds. You don't need any special skills or equipment to get started, just a willingness to give it a try.

4. Is it normal to struggle with racing thoughts during meditation?

Yes, it's entirely normal to have a racing mind during meditation, especially when you're just starting. The key is not to judge yourself for it. Simply acknowledge the thoughts and gently bring your focus back to your chosen point of meditation, whether it's your breath, a mantra, or a visual object.

5. Can mindfulness and meditation be done together with other treatments for depression?

Yes, they can be complementary to other treatments for depression. Many therapists incorporate mindfulness and meditation into their treatment plans, and they can be used alongside medication as well. Always consult with a healthcare professional to determine the best approach for your specific needs.

In the hustle and bustle of modern life, depression can often creep in like an uninvited guest. But with the power of mindfulness and meditation, you can take charge of your mental well-being. Understanding mindfulness and meditation for managing depression is like having a secret weapon in your arsenal—a way to find peace and tranquility in even the stormiest of times.

So, if you're feeling overwhelmed by the daily grind or struggling with the weight of depression, why not give mindfulness and meditation a try? Start small, be patient with yourself, and remember that you're not alone on this journey. With a little mindfulness and meditation, you can find your way back to a happier, healthier you. Understanding mindfulness and meditation for managing depression is your ticket to a brighter future.

Chapter 12

The Role of Nutrition and Exercise in Mental Health

The right combination of nutrition and exercise, puts you on a path to a happier, healthier mind

In the hustle and bustle of modern life, we often overlook the profound connection between what we eat, how we move, and the state of our mental well-being. While it's no secret that nutrition and exercise are crucial for physical health, their impact on mental health is equally significant, if not more so. Learn the fascinating realm of how what you put on your plate and how you get moving can drastically affect your mental state. So, let's put on our mental workout gear and explore "The Role of Nutrition and Exercise in Mental Health!"

Understanding the Mind-Body Connection

To fully appreciate the role of nutrition and exercise in mental health, it's vital to understand the intricate mind-body connection. Our brain, the command center of our body, isn't a solitary entity but closely linked to the rest of our system. This interconnectedness means that the food we consume and the physical activities we engage in directly impact our mental well-being.

How Nutrition Influences Your Mental State

Ever heard the phrase "you are what you eat"? Well, when it comes to your brain, this saying hits the bullseye. The brain requires a variety of nutrients to function optimally, including:

Omega-3 Fatty Acids: Found in fatty fish like salmon and walnuts, these healthy fats are essential for brain health. They help build brain cell membranes and reduce inflammation, which can lead to improved mood and cognitive function.

Antioxidants: Fruits and vegetables like blueberries, spinach, and kale are packed with antioxidants. These compounds protect your brain from oxidative stress and may reduce the risk of mental decline.

Complex Carbohydrates: Foods like whole grains, beans, and lentils provide a steady supply of glucose to the brain. This helps maintain focus and stabilizes mood.

Protein: Amino acids from protein-rich foods help produce neurotransmitters like serotonin and dopamine, which are key players in regulating mood.

The Gut-Brain Connection

Believe it or not, your gut health is closely intertwined with your mental health. The gut-brain axis is a complex network of communication between the digestive system and the brain. A healthy gut microbiome, which can be nurtured through a balanced diet, is associated with reduced symptoms of anxiety and depression.

Blood Sugar Rollercoaster

Ever experienced a sudden mood swing after indulging in sugary snacks? Blame it on the blood sugar rollercoaster! Foods high in sugar can lead to rapid spikes and crashes in blood sugar levels, which can wreak havoc on your mood and energy levels.

The Impact of Exercise on Mental Health:

The Feel-Good Hormones: Endorphins

You've probably heard of the "runner's high," but you don't have to be a marathoner to experience it. Exercise, whether it's a brisk walk, a yoga session, or a dance class, triggers the release of endorphins. These natural mood lifters can help combat stress, anxiety, and depression.

Stress Reduction and Cortisol

Life's stressors can take a toll on your mental health, but regular exercise can be your secret weapon against stress. Physical activity reduces the production of cortisol, a stress hormone, while increasing the release of feel-good neurotransmitters like endorphins and serotonin.

Improved Sleep

Sleep is the unsung hero of mental well-being. Exercise can improve both the quality and duration of your slumber, ensuring you wake up feeling refreshed and ready to tackle the day. Poor sleep, on the other hand, is closely linked to mood disorders.

Nutrition and Mental Health: What to Eat for a Happy Mind

Now that we've established the connection between nutrition and mental health, let's get down to the nitty-gritty of what you should include in your diet to boost your mood and keep your mental health in check!

The Mood-Boosting Menu

Fatty Fish

Salmon, mackerel, and sardines are your go-to sources of omega-3 fatty acids. These fish are like little brain powerhouses that can enhance your mood and cognitive function. Try to incorporate them into your diet at least twice a week.

Colorful Fruits and Vegetables

The vibrant colors of fruits and veggies aren't just visually appealing; they're loaded with antioxidants that protect your brain cells from damage. Aim for a rainbow on your plate to ensure you get a wide range of nutrients.

Whole Grains

Opt for whole grains like brown rice, quinoa, and oats instead of refined grains. They release energy slowly, preventing those energy crashes that can lead to mood swings.

Lean Protein

Chicken, turkey, tofu, and beans are excellent sources of protein. They provide the amino acids your brain needs to produce neurotransmitters that regulate your mood.

Probiotic Foods

Cultivate a healthy gut microbiome by including yogurt, kefir, sauerkraut, and kimchi in your diet. A happy gut often leads to a happier mind.

Nuts and Seeds

Almonds, walnuts, and flaxseeds are rich in nutrients that support brain health. They're also great for snacking when you need an energy boost.

Hydration

Don't forget to drink plenty of water! Even mild dehydration can affect your mood and cognitive function.

What to Limit or Avoid

Sugar and Refined Carbs

Minimize your intake of sugary snacks, sugary drinks, and refined carbohydrates like white bread and pastries. They can lead to rapid blood sugar fluctuations and mood swings.

Processed Foods

Processed foods often contain unhealthy trans fats and excessive sodium. These can negatively impact both physical and mental health.

Alcohol and Caffeine

While the occasional glass of wine or cup of coffee is fine, excessive alcohol and caffeine consumption can disrupt sleep patterns and exacerbate anxiety.

Exercise and Mental Health: Get Moving for a Happier Mind

Now, let's break a sweat and explore how different types of exercises can elevate your mental well-being. Remember, it's not about becoming a fitness guru overnight; even small, regular doses of physical activity can make a significant difference.

Cardiovascular Exercises

Running and Jogging

Running isn't just a great workout for your body; it's a fantastic mental health booster too! The rhythmic motion and steady pace can clear your mind and reduce stress.

Cycling

Whether you're pedaling through scenic routes or spinning in the gym, cycling is a low-impact exercise that can improve your mood and increase energy levels.

Dancing

Crank up your favorite tunes and dance like no one's watching! Dancing is not only fun but also an excellent way to release those endorphins and boost your self-esteem.

Strength Training

Weightlifting

Lifting weights can do wonders for your confidence and body image. As you get stronger physically, you're likely to feel stronger mentally too.

Bodyweight Exercises

You don't need fancy equipment to get fit. Push-ups, squats, and planks can all be done at home and are great for building both muscle and mental resilience.

Mind-Body Exercises

Yoga

Yoga combines physical postures with mindfulness and deep breathing. It's a holistic practice that can reduce stress and promote mental clarity.

Pilates

Pilates focuses on core strength and flexibility. It can help improve posture and alleviate back pain, which can have a positive impact on your mental well-being.

Tai Chi

This gentle martial art is like a moving meditation. Tai Chi can improve balance, reduce anxiety, and promote a sense of inner peace.

Team Sports and Social Activities

Basketball, Soccer, or Volleyball

Joining a sports team is an excellent way to stay active and socialize. The camaraderie and competition can boost your mood and self-esteem.

Group Fitness Classes

Whether it's Zumba, spinning, or HIIT classes, exercising in a group setting can be motivating and foster a sense of belonging.

Answering Your Burning Questions

Can I improve my mental health solely through diet and exercise?

While nutrition and exercise play pivotal roles in mental health, they are not standalone solutions. A holistic approach that may include therapy, mindfulness practices, and medication, if necessary, is often recommended for severe mental health conditions.

How long should I exercise each day to reap mental health benefits?

Aim for at least 30 minutes of moderate-intensity exercise most days of the week. However, even shorter bouts of exercise can provide immediate mood-enhancing effects.

Are there specific diets that are best for mental health?

No single diet works for everyone, but a balanced diet rich in whole foods, as mentioned earlier, is generally beneficial for mental health. It's also essential to tailor your diet to your individual needs and preferences.

What if I don't enjoy traditional forms of exercise?

That's okay! Find physical activities you genuinely enjoy, whether it's dancing, hiking, gardening, or even playing a musical instrument. The key is to stay active in a way that brings you joy.

How quickly can I expect to see improvements in my mental health through nutrition and exercise?

The timeline varies from person to person. Some individuals experience immediate mood improvements after a single workout or a healthy meal, while others may take several weeks to notice significant changes. Consistency is key.

The choices you make about what you eat and how you move can profoundly impact your mood, stress levels, and overall mental health. So, let's recap the key takeaways:

Nutrition: Opt for brain-boosting foods like fatty fish, colorful fruits and veggies, whole grains, lean protein, and probiotic-rich options. Limit or avoid sugar, refined carbs, and processed foods.

Exercise: Incorporate cardiovascular, strength training, and mind-body exercises into your routine. Choose activities you enjoy to make staying active a sustainable part of your life.

Remember that mental health is a journey, and there's no one-size-fits-all approach. Be patient with yourself, seek support when needed, and celebrate the small victories along the way. With the right combination of nutrition and exercise, you can embark on a path to a happier, healthier mind—one step (and one bite) at a time!

Chapter 13

Reconnecting with Your Passions and Purpose when Dealing with Depression

Rekindling your passions is like finding a compass in the wilderness of depression

Depression can be a relentless adversary, casting a shadow over even the most vibrant aspects of our lives. It saps our energy, dims our enthusiasm, and leaves us feeling adrift in a sea of hopelessness. But what if there was a lifeboat to rescue us from the depths of despair? What if we could reconnect with our passions and purpose, using them as beacons to guide us through the stormy seas of depression? Embark on a journey to explore how you can reignite that inner fire, find your sense of purpose, and reclaim your zest for life.

Unveiling the Fog of Depression

Depression, like a dense fog, can shroud our minds and obscure our sense of self. It blurs the vivid colors of our interests and aspirations, making everything appear gray and lifeless. Before we can embark on the path to rekindling our passions and purpose, we must first understand the nature of depression and its impact on our lives.

The Weight of Depression

Depression is more than just feeling sad or having a bad day. It's a persistent and pervasive mental health condition that affects millions of people worldwide. The weight of depression can feel crushing, as if a dark cloud hovers over your every thought and action. It's important to recognize that depression is not a sign of weakness; it's an illness that requires attention and care.

The Erosion of Passion and Purpose

One of the most insidious aspects of depression is its ability to erode our passions and rob us of our sense of purpose. It's like a thief in the night, stealing away the very things that once brought us joy and fulfillment. When we're in the throes of depression, it can be challenging to remember what it's like to be passionate about something or to feel that our lives have purpose.

The Isolation Trap

Depression often leads to isolation, as we withdraw from social interactions and activities we once enjoyed. This isolation can further exacerbate our sense of purposelessness, as we feel disconnected from the world around us. Breaking free from this trap is a crucial step in the journey to reconnecting with your passions and purpose.

Finding Your North Star: Reconnecting with Your Passions

Rekindling your passions is like finding a compass in the wilderness of depression. Your passions are the things that ignite your soul, the activities that make your heart race with excitement. Here's how you can start rediscovering and nurturing those passions:

1. Reflect on Your Past

Think back to the activities or hobbies that used to bring you immense joy. What were you passionate about before depression cast its shadow? It could be anything from painting and hiking to cooking or playing a musical instrument. Make a list of these activities and memories.

2. Start Small

When dealing with depression, it's essential to start small. The prospect of diving headfirst into a long-lost passion may feel overwhelming. Begin by dedicating just a few minutes each day to one of the activities on your list. The key is to reacquaint yourself gradually.

3. Embrace Curiosity

Sometimes, depression can make us feel as though we've lost touch with our interests entirely. In such cases, embrace curiosity as your guide. Explore new activities and experiences, even if they seem unrelated to your previous passions. You might stumble upon something that reignites your inner spark.

4. Seek Support

Reconnecting with your passions doesn't have to be a solitary journey. Reach out to friends or support groups that share your interests. Connecting with others who have a similar passion can provide motivation and a sense of belonging.

5. Be Patient

Remember, progress may be slow, and setbacks are natural. Be patient with yourself and acknowledge that the path to rediscovering your passions may be filled with twists and turns. The important thing is to keep moving forward, even if it's at a snail's pace.

Rekindling Your Purpose: A Beacon in the Darkness

Purpose is the lighthouse that guides us through the stormy seas of depression. It gives our lives meaning and direction, helping us navigate even the darkest of nights. Here's how you can begin the process of reconnecting with your sense of purpose:

1. Identify Your Values

Your values are the core principles that define who you are and what you believe in. Take some time to reflect on your values. What matters most to you? Is it creativity, kindness, adventure, or something else entirely? Understanding your values can provide clarity about your purpose.

2. Set Meaningful Goals

Having goals can infuse your life with purpose. Start by setting small, achievable goals that align with your values. These could be as simple as volunteering for a cause you care about, learning a new skill, or reconnecting with an old friend.

3. Find Your "Why"

Simon Sinek famously said, "Start with why." Delve deep into the reasons behind your actions and choices. Ask yourself why you want to pursue a particular goal or engage in a specific activity. Understanding your "why" can reveal your underlying purpose.

4. Give Back

Contributing to the well-being of others can be a powerful source of purpose. Consider ways in which you can make a positive impact on your community or the world at large. Even small acts of kindness can reignite your sense of purpose.

5. Embrace Change

Your sense of purpose may evolve over time, and that's perfectly normal. Embrace change and be open to reevaluating your goals and values as you grow. Your purpose is not set in stone; it can adapt and expand along with you.

Can I reconnect with my passions and purpose even if I've been battling depression for years?

Absolutely! While it may take time and effort, reconnecting with your passions and purpose is possible, no matter how long you've been dealing with depression. Remember that progress is a journey, not a destination.

What if I don't know what my passions or purpose are anymore?

It's common to feel lost in this regard, especially when depression has clouded your vision. Start by exploring new activities and being open to curiosity. Sometimes, your passions and purpose can reveal themselves through unexpected experiences.

Is professional help necessary when dealing with depression and trying to reconnect with passions and purpose?

Professional help, such as therapy or counseling, can be immensely beneficial when dealing with depression. A mental health professional can provide guidance, support, and strategies tailored to your specific needs. Don't hesitate to seek help if you need it.

What if I face setbacks or lose motivation along the way?

Setbacks are a natural part of any journey, especially when dealing with depression. It's essential to be patient with yourself and practice self-compassion. If you lose motivation, try reaching out to friends, support groups, or a therapist for encouragement.

Can reconnecting with passions and purpose cure depression?

Reconnecting with your passions and purpose can be a valuable component of managing depression, but it may not be a cure on its own. It's crucial to pursue a holistic approach to mental health, which may include therapy, medication, self-care, and a support system.

Illuminating the Path Forward

Depression may cast a shadow, but within that darkness lies the potential for rediscovery. Reconnecting with your passions and purpose when dealing with depression is a journey worth embarking upon. It's a path illuminated by the sparks of your interests and the guiding light of your purpose.

Remember, you are not alone on this journey. Reach out to friends, family, or professionals who can support you along the way. Embrace curiosity, be patient with yourself, and allow your passions and purpose to lead you back to a life filled with color, meaning, and vitality.

So, take that first step today—embrace the challenge, find your passions, and let your purpose shine as a beacon of hope in the midst of the storm. You have the power to reconnect with your passions and purpose, and in doing so, you can find the strength to conquer depression and reclaim your zest for life. It's a journey worth taking, and the destination is a brighter, more fulfilling future.

Reconnecting with Your Passions and Purpose when dealing with depression—it's not just a possibility; it's your path to rediscovery and renewal.

Chapter 14

Managing Setbacks in Depression Battle

Understanding what you're up against is the first step toward conquering it.

A re you in the midst of a relentless battle with depression, facing setbacks that seem insurmountable? Well, you're not alone! Managing setbacks in your depression journey can feel like a never-ending rollercoaster of emotions, but fear not; there are ways to navigate this challenging terrain and emerge stronger on the other side. The chapter discusses strategies and insights on handling setbacks while fighting depression. From understanding the nature of setbacks to practical tips and real-life stories, we've got you covered.

Understanding Setbacks in Depression

Before we dive into the strategies for managing setbacks, it's crucial to grasp the nature of these ups and downs in your depression battle. Understanding what you're up against is the first step toward conquering it.

What Are Setbacks in Depression?

Setbacks in depression refer to those moments when it feels like all your progress has been erased, and you're back at square one, or worse. These setbacks can manifest in various forms:

Emotional Slumps: You might suddenly find yourself overwhelmed by sadness, anxiety, or despair, even if you were doing well before.

Loss of Interest: Hobbies or activities that once brought you joy might suddenly lose their appeal, leaving you feeling empty.

Fatigue and Apathy: Daily tasks become Herculean challenges, and you may feel utterly indifferent toward your responsibilities.

Social Withdrawal: The desire to isolate yourself from friends and family may intensify during setbacks.

Negative Self-Talk: Setbacks often come hand in hand with a barrage of self-critical and pessimistic thoughts.

Why Do Setbacks Happen?

Understanding the triggers behind setbacks is as crucial as recognizing their symptoms. Here are some common reasons why setbacks occur:

Life Events: Stressful situations, such as the loss of a loved one, job problems, or relationship difficulties, can trigger setbacks.

Chemical Imbalances: Depression is often linked to imbalances in brain chemicals, and these imbalances can fluctuate, leading to setbacks.

Lack of Consistency: Inconsistent self-care routines, like irregular sleep patterns or poor nutrition, can contribute to setbacks.

Overexertion: Pushing yourself too hard to maintain a facade of normalcy can exhaust your mental and emotional resources, leading to setbacks.

Unrealistic Expectations: Setting overly ambitious goals or expecting instant results can set you up for disappointment and setbacks.

Strategies for Managing Setbacks

Now that we have a clearer picture of what setbacks in depression are, let's explore some practical strategies to manage them effectively. Remember, there's no one-size-fits-all approach, so feel free to mix and match these strategies to find what works best for you.

1. Embrace Self-Compassion

In the midst of a setback, it's easy to beat yourself up for not being 'strong enough' or 'better' by now. However, self-compassion is the antidote to self-criticism. Treat yourself as you would a dear friend going through a tough time:

Practice Self-Talk: Replace negative self-talk with kind and understanding words. Remind yourself that setbacks are a part of the journey.

Self-Care Rituals: Engage in self-care activities that nourish your body and soul, whether it's a warm bath, a good book, or a meditation session.

Seek Support: Don't hesitate to reach out to friends, family, or a therapist who can provide the support and compassion you need.

2. Set Realistic Goals

During your depression battle, it's essential to set achievable goals. When setbacks occur, it's often because the expectations placed upon yourself are too high. Here's how to set and adjust your goals:

Break It Down: Divide your goals into smaller, manageable steps. This makes progress less daunting and setbacks less devastating.

Flexible Goals: Be open to adjusting your goals when necessary. Sometimes, your depression journey might take unexpected turns, and that's okay.

Celebrate Small Wins: Acknowledge and celebrate every little achievement, no matter how minor it may seem. Each step forward is a victory.

3. Maintain a Support System

You don't have to face setbacks in your depression battle alone. Building and maintaining a strong support system is crucial for weathering the storm:

Reach Out: Don't isolate yourself during setbacks. Reach out to friends or family members who understand your struggles.

Online Communities: Join online forums or support groups where you can connect with others who are going through similar experiences.

Therapy: Consider therapy or counseling as a consistent source of support and guidance throughout your journey.

4. Keep a Journal

Journaling can be a powerful tool for managing setbacks in depression. It allows you to track your emotions, identify patterns, and gain insights into your mental health:

Daily Reflections: Dedicate a few minutes each day to jot down your thoughts and feelings. This can help you pinpoint triggers and recognize early warning signs of setbacks.

Gratitude Journal: In addition to venting your emotions, maintain a gratitude journal to focus on the positive aspects of your life, no matter how small.

Goal Tracker: Use your journal to track your progress toward your goals. Seeing your achievements in writing can boost your motivation.

5. Seek Professional Help

While self-help strategies are valuable, it's essential to acknowledge when you need professional assistance. Therapists, psychiatrists, and mental health experts can provide specialized guidance and treatments tailored to your needs.

Therapy: Cognitive-behavioral therapy (CBT) and dialectical behavior therapy (DBT) are effective for managing depression and setbacks.

Medication: In some cases, medication prescribed by a psychiatrist can help stabilize mood and alleviate symptoms.

Supportive Services: Explore additional resources such as support groups or community mental health services.

Real-Life Stories: Triumph over Setbacks

To truly understand the art of managing setbacks in the depression battle, let's draw inspiration from real individuals who have faced setbacks and emerged stronger:

Story 1: Rebecca's Resilience

Rebecca, a 32-year-old marketing professional, battled depression for years. Her setbacks often occurred when work stress and personal life challenges collided. During one particularly difficult period, she sought therapy and began practicing self-compassion.

"I used to blame myself for not being 'normal,'" Rebecca shared. "But my therapist helped me understand that setbacks happen to everyone, not just me. It's okay to have bad days."

Rebecca gradually implemented self-care rituals into her routine, including yoga and meditation. Over time, she discovered the power of setting small, achievable goals.

"Each day, I'd set one goal, like taking a 10-minute walk or sending a text to a friend," she said. "These small victories added up, and I realized that even on my worst days, I was making progress."

Story 2: Anderson's Support System

Anderson, a 45-year-old teacher, faced setbacks during his depression journey, often triggered by seasonal changes and family stress. He emphasized the importance of seeking support:

"I used to bottle up my feelings, thinking I could handle it alone," Anderson admitted. "But it was isolating and made the setbacks feel even more overwhelming."

Anderson reached out to a therapist who introduced him to mindfulness techniques and helped him build a support network of friends and family members. This network became his lifeline during setbacks.

"Having people who genuinely care about you and understand what you're going through is priceless," Anderson said. "They remind you that you're not alone in this battle."

Story 3: Lucy's Journaling Journey

Lucy, a 28-year-old artist, turned to journaling as a way to manage her setbacks. Her depression often manifested as creative blocks and self-doubt. She shared her journaling experience:

"At first, I thought journaling was just writing down my feelings," Lucy said. "But it became a tool for self-discovery. I started to see patterns in my emotions and behavior."

Lucy's journal became a space for daily reflections, goal tracking, and gratitude lists. Through this practice, she discovered that setbacks were opportunities for growth.

"When I hit a creative roadblock, instead of getting frustrated, I'd write about it," she explained. "It helped me understand my creative process better and find new inspiration."

How long do setbacks in depression typically last?

Setbacks in depression vary in duration from person to person. Some may experience brief setbacks lasting a few days, while others might endure longer episodes. The key is to focus on self-care and seek support during these challenging times.

Are setbacks a sign of personal failure?

No, setbacks in depression are not indicative of personal failure. Depression is a complex condition influenced by various factors, including genetics and life experiences. Setbacks are a natural part of the journey and should be viewed as opportunities for growth.

Can setbacks be prevented altogether?

While it's challenging to prevent setbacks entirely, managing your mental health through self-care, therapy, and support systems can reduce their frequency and intensity. The goal is not to eliminate setbacks but to equip yourself with the tools to navigate them successfully.

Is it okay to seek professional help for setbacks?

Absolutely! Seeking professional help, such as therapy or medication, is a valid and effective approach to managing setbacks in depression. Mental health experts can provide tailored strategies and support to help you overcome challenges.

Managing setbacks in the depression battle is an ongoing process that requires patience, self-compassion, and resilience. By understanding the nature of setbacks, setting realistic goals, maintaining a support system, journaling, and, when needed, seeking professional help, you can navigate the rollercoaster of emotions with greater confidence.

Remember, setbacks are not a sign of weakness or failure; they are part of the journey toward recovery. Real-life stories of individuals like Rebecca, Anderson, and Lucy remind us that triumph over setbacks is possible. With the right strategies and support, you can emerge from setbacks even stronger, ready to continue your battle against depression.

So, as you face the ups and downs of your depression journey, hold onto the knowledge that managing setbacks is not just about surviving but thriving, one step at a time.

You've got this, and there's a brighter tomorrow waiting for you!

Chapter 15

Celebrating Milestones: Recognizing Your Progress

Celebrating small milestones is crucial because it boosts your motivation and reinforces your commitment to your goals.

I n the journey of life, we all encounter milestones, both big and small. These moments mark significant achievements, and they have the power to shape our motivations, aspirations, and ultimately, our success. Celebrating milestones can have on our motivation levels and how it can drive us to achieve even greater heights.

The Brain's Reward System

Our brains are wired to seek rewards and positive reinforcement. When you recognize progress, you trigger the release of dopamine, the "feel-good" neurotransmitter. This not only makes you feel happy but also encourages you to keep moving forward. It's like your brain's way of saying, "Keep up the good work!"

The Pitfalls of Neglecting Progress

Now, imagine for a moment that you never acknowledge your progress. What happens then?

Demotivation: Without positive reinforcement, you're likely to feel demotivated and may even give up on your goals.

Burnout: Constantly chasing distant milestones without recognizing your achievements can lead to burnout. It's like running a marathon without ever stopping for water.

Low Self-Esteem: Neglecting progress can erode your self-esteem, leaving you feeling unworthy and incapable.

Understanding the Significance of Milestones

Defining Milestones

Before we explore how milestones boost motivation, let's establish what milestones are. Milestones are specific, measurable points in our journey that indicate progress or achievement. They can be personal or professional, ranging from completing a project ahead of schedule to hitting a fitness goal. Essentially, milestones are the markers that define our path to success.

The Psychological Impact

Milestones play a pivotal role in psychology, and understanding this impact is key to unlocking their motivational potential. When we set and achieve milestones, our brains release a surge of dopamine, the "feel-good" neurotransmitter. This rush of positive emotion is a powerful motivator, encouraging us to strive for more milestones and accomplishments.

How Celebrating Milestones Boosts Motivation

Reinforcing Success

One of the most significant ways celebrating milestones boosts motivation is by reinforcing our sense of success.

When we acknowledge and celebrate our achievements, we remind ourselves that we are capable of progress and success. This reinforcement acts as a powerful motivator to continue working towards our goals.

Building Confidence

Confidence is a cornerstone of motivation. When we celebrate milestones, we build our confidence in our abilities. Each milestone achieved serves as evidence of our competence, and this self-assurance fuels our motivation to take on more significant challenges.

Providing a Sense of Direction

Milestones also provide a clear sense of direction. They break down long-term goals into manageable steps. This clear path allows us to focus our efforts and maintain a sense of purpose, ultimately boosting our motivation to reach the next milestone in our journey.

Cultivating a Growth Mindset

Celebrating milestones fosters a growth mindset—a belief that abilities and intelligence can be developed through dedication and hard work. This mindset shift is crucial for long-term motivation, as it encourages us to view setbacks as opportunities for growth rather than as failures.

Practical Ways to Celebrate Milestones

Reflect and Appreciate

Taking time to reflect on your achievements is a simple yet powerful way to celebrate milestones. Write down what you've accomplished, how it makes you feel, and the steps you took to get there. This self-appreciation reinforces the positive emotions associated with success.

Reward Yourself

Treat yourself when you reach a milestone. Whether it's indulging in your favorite dessert, enjoying a relaxing day off, or buying yourself a small gift, rewards can serve as powerful motivators and make your journey towards your goals more enjoyable.

Share Your Success

Sharing your milestones with friends, family, or colleagues not only celebrates your achievements but also strengthens your support network. Their encouragement and validation can further boost your motivation.

Set New Goals

After celebrating a milestone, it's essential to set new goals. This keeps the momentum going and ensures that you have a constant source of motivation driving you forward.

Real-Life Examples of Milestone Celebrations

Professional Milestones

Job Promotion: Celebrate a promotion by sharing your accomplishment with coworkers, and treat yourself to a nice dinner or weekend getaway.

Project Completion: After successfully completing a challenging project, acknowledge your hard work and consider taking a day off to relax and recharge.

Personal Milestones

Fitness Goals: When you hit a fitness milestone, such as running a certain distance or achieving a specific weight, reward yourself with new workout gear or a spa day.

Learning Achievements: If you've acquired a new skill or completed a course, celebrate by sharing your achievement with peers and setting your sights on the next learning opportunity.

Maintaining Motivation through Milestones

While celebrating milestones is a powerful motivator, it's essential to maintain that motivation over the long term. Here are some strategies to keep the momentum going:

Stay Consistent

Consistency is key to staying motivated. Continue setting and celebrating milestones regularly, even after achieving major goals. This keeps your motivation levels high and your focus sharp.

Track Your Progress

Keep a record of your milestones and progress. This visual representation of your journey serves as a constant reminder of how far you've come and where you're headed.

Embrace Challenges

Don't shy away from challenges. Embrace them as opportunities to achieve new milestones and grow as an individual. Challenges are the building blocks of personal and professional development.

Creative Ways to Celebrate Your Achievements

Celebrating milestones doesn't have to be a routine affair. Get creative and infuse your celebrations with personality. Here are some innovative ideas for making your achievements memorable.

Personal Celebrations

- *Write a Gratitude Journal:* Document your journey, including the milestones you've conquered. Reflecting on your progress can be a rewarding experience.
- *Treat Yourself:* Buy that item you've been eyeing, indulge in your favorite dessert, or take a spa day.
- *Travel Adventures:* Plan a getaway to celebrate significant milestones. Exploring new places can be a great way to reward yourself.

Social Celebrations

- *Host a Gathering:* Invite friends and family for a milestone-themed party. Share your achievements and bask in their congratulatory cheers.
- *Give Back:* Celebrate by volunteering or donating to a cause you're passionate about. It's a way to spread the joy.
- *Share on Social Media:* Let the world know about your accomplishments. It can inspire others and create a positive ripple effect.

Professional Celebrations

Team Acknowledgment: In a group setting, recognize your team's milestones collectively. It fosters a sense of unity and achievement.

Personal Growth Workshop: Invest in your professional development as a reward for achieving significant milestones.

Milestone Awards: Some social groups have milestone awards programs in place. If not, suggest implementing one.

Overcoming Challenges along the Way

While the journey to your goals is exciting, it's not without its challenges. Recognizing and celebrating milestones can also help you navigate the hurdles effectively.

Dealing with Setbacks

Even the most successful journeys have their setbacks. Instead of dwelling on them, treat setbacks as opportunities to learn and grow. When you eventually overcome these obstacles, it becomes a milestone in itself, worthy of celebration.

Milestones are not just markers of success; they are powerful motivators that can propel us towards greater achievements. By celebrating milestones, we reinforce our successes, boost our confidence, and cultivate a growth mindset. Whether in our personal or professional lives, the act of celebrating milestones keeps us on track, provides a sense of direction, and ultimately leads to more significant accomplishments.

So, as you embark on your journey towards your goals, remember the importance of celebrating each milestone along the way. It's not just a celebration of the past; it's an investment in your future success.

Why should I celebrate small milestones?

Celebrating small milestones is crucial because it boosts your motivation and reinforces your commitment to your goals. It's these smaller victories that pave the way for more significant achievements.

How can I make milestone celebrations more memorable?

Get creative! Personal celebrations can involve journaling, treats, or travel. Social celebrations can include gatherings or giving back, while professional celebrations might involve team recognition or personal growth workshops.

What if I face setbacks on my journey?

Setbacks are a natural part of any journey. Instead of being discouraged, treat them as opportunities for growth. Overcoming setbacks can become significant milestones in themselves.

Is it essential to celebrate long-term milestones as well?

Yes, celebrating long-term milestones is crucial because they provide a sense of direction and purpose. Balancing both short-term and long-term celebrations ensures sustained progress.

How does milestone recognition affect motivation?

Milestone recognition triggers the release of dopamine in the brain, enhancing your mood and strengthening your commitment to your goals. It keeps you motivated and focused on your journey.

Chapter 16

Embracing a Brighter Future: Your Path to Wholeness

Setbacks are part of the journey, embrace them as opportunities to learn and grow

Are you tired of the daily grind, the feeling that life is passing you by? Do you yearn for something more, something that will light up your world with purpose and fulfillment? In this ever-changing world, many of us find ourselves on a quest for wholeness and a brighter future.

But fear not! Embracing a brighter future and finding your path to wholeness is not some elusive dream. It's a tangible reality waiting for you to seize.

Unveiling the Concept of Wholeness

What is Wholeness, Anyway?

First things first, let's clear the fog surrounding the term "wholeness." What does it even mean? Well, in the context we're talking about, wholeness refers to a state of completeness and inner harmony. It's about feeling fulfilled, content, and connected to your true self. It's like putting together all the pieces of a puzzle that is you!

The Importance of Wholeness

Why should you care about achieving wholeness? Ah, that's the million-dollar question! Here's the deal:

Wholeness leads to happiness: When you're whole, you're more likely to experience joy and satisfaction in life.

Better relationships: You'll form deeper connections with others when you're in tune with yourself.

Improved mental health: Wholeness can reduce stress, anxiety, and depression.

Enhanced resilience: You'll bounce back from setbacks with greater strength and resilience.

So, embracing a brighter future through wholeness isn't just a fluffy concept—it's a game-changer!

Your Path to Wholeness

1. *Self-Discovery:* Know Thyself

The journey to wholeness begins with self-discovery. You can't embrace a brighter future if you don't know what truly lights you up. Here's how to get started:

- Reflect on your passions and interests. What makes your heart race with excitement?
- Identify your strengths and weaknesses. What are you good at, and where do you need improvement?
- Explore your values and beliefs. What do you stand for? What matters most to you?
- Seek feedback from trusted friends and family. Sometimes, they see things you might have missed.

2. Set Clear Goals

Once you've got a better grip on who you are, it's time to set some goals. But hold on, don't just scribble down random wishes! Be specific and strategic:

- Create SMART goals (Specific, Measurable, Achievable, Relevant, Time-bound).
- Break down your big goals into smaller, manageable steps.
- Keep a journal to track your progress and celebrate small wins along the way.
- Embrace flexibility—your goals can evolve as you do.

3. Embrace Change

Change is inevitable on the path to wholeness. Instead of resisting it, embrace it like an old friend. Change can:

- Lead to personal growth and self-improvement.
- Open up new opportunities you never imagined.
- Challenge your comfort zone and push you to reach your full potential.
- Remember, it's not about changing who you are; it's about evolving into the best version of yourself!

4. Cultivate Mindfulness

In our hectic lives, it's easy to get lost in the chaos. That's where mindfulness comes in. It's all about being present in the moment, and it can help you:

- Reduce stress and anxiety.
- Improve focus and concentration.
- Enhance self-awareness and emotional regulation.
- Strengthen your connection with yourself and others.

So, start practicing mindfulness through techniques like meditation, deep breathing, or even a daily gratitude journal.

5. Seek Support and Guidance

Embracing a brighter future and achieving wholeness isn't a solo mission. It's perfectly okay to seek support and guidance along the way:

- Connect with a mentor or coach who can provide valuable insights and encouragement.
- Build a support network of friends and family who believe in your journey.
- Consider therapy or counseling if you're facing deep-rooted challenges.

- Remember, asking for help is a sign of strength, not weakness.

Can anyone achieve wholeness?

Absolutely! Wholeness is attainable for everyone willing to embark on the journey of self-discovery and personal growth.

How long does it take to achieve wholeness?

The timeline varies for each person. It depends on your starting point, goals, and commitment to the journey. Some see significant changes in months, while for others, it might take years.

What if I face setbacks or obstacles?

Setbacks are part of the journey. Embrace them as opportunities to learn and grow. Seek support when needed, and keep moving forward.

Is it too late to start my journey to wholeness?

It's never too late! No matter your age or circumstances, the path to wholeness is open to everyone.

Can I achieve wholeness while maintaining my current job and responsibilities?

Absolutely! Wholeness can be integrated into your daily life. It's about finding balance and aligning your choices with your values and passions.

Embracing a brighter future and achieving wholeness is within your reach. It all starts with self-discovery, setting clear goals, embracing change, cultivating mindfulness, and seeking support and guidance.

So, what are you waiting for? Take the first step on your path to wholeness today. Remember, it's not about reaching some distant destination; it's about savoring the journey, one step at a time. Your brighter future is waiting to unfold, and it begins with you!

---------------- I Wish you Success -----------------